C(

Intermittent Fasting 101: *The Ultimate Guide to Losing Weight & Feeling Great with an IF Diet*

June 2014

SJ

www.IgnoreLimits.com

Disclaimer

The information provided in this book is designed to provide helpful information on the subjects discussed. This book is not meant to be used, nor should it be used, to diagnose or treat any medical condition. For diagnosis or treatment of any medical problem, consult your own physician. The publisher and author are not responsible for any specific health or allergy needs that may require medical supervision and are not liable for any damages or negative consequences from any treatment, action, application or preparation, to any person reading or following the information in this book. References are provided for informational purposes only and do not constitute endorsement of any websites or other sources. Readers should be aware that the websites listed in this book may   change.

I recommend consulting a doctor to assess and/or identify any health related issues prior to making any dramatic changes to your diet and/or exercise regime.

Contents

Introduction

I want to thank you and congratulate you for downloading the book, *"Intermittent Fasting 101: The Ultimate Guide to Losing Weight & Feeling Great with an IF Diet"*.

This book contains proven steps and strategies on how to lose weight and gain muscle through intermittent fasting. It also contains new research and studies done to test the effectiveness of the approach. Through this book you will discover how people lose weight in a natural way without depriving themselves of the foods they like. The pros and cons of IF are also discussed in detail. If you want to learn more and understand intermittent fasting further, this book is perfect for you.

Thanks again for downloading this book, I hope you enjoy it!

About the Author

Hi there, I'm SJ.

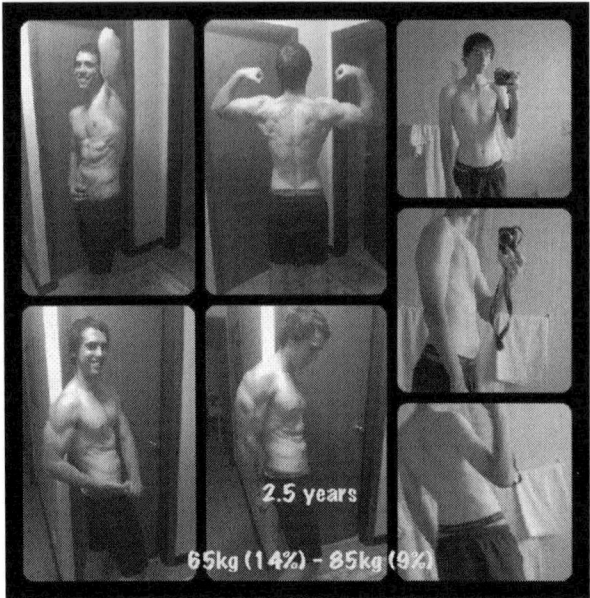

My Story thus far

I graduated high school with no direction in life and a frail physique weighing in at a mere 135lbs, I was unhappy with essentially all aspects of my life.

Then one day it all changed.

I finally realized that I am the only one to blame, when I looked in the mirror that day I realized that I had connected the dots, that the life I was currently living was the end result of all the decisions I had made leading up to that day. Every time I chose to play Xbox instead of hitting the gym, every time I slept in instead of waking up to study and make something of myself lead me to where I currently was.

From that day forward I took ownership of my actions, I began to hit the gym multiple times per week, I applied for scholarships and successfully had my tuition paid for in full, I read books, TONS of books on everything to do with the mind and body.

It was all on me.

My results?

I transformed my body from a skinny fat 135lbs with 18% body fat to a solid 192lbs at 9% body fat.

I became qualified in a field I was passionate about.

I learnt a plethora of new information on dieting and fitness by reading and applying what I read, to find out what does work and what doesn't work, because as I'm sure you've noticed the health and fitness industry is full of non-sense claims and BS. I found out what was true and what worked for me and applied that knowledge.

And you bet I had fun during the whole process.

Bonus Content

As a token of my appreciation, I'd like to give you access to my exclusive bonus content.

Here's what you're about to receive...

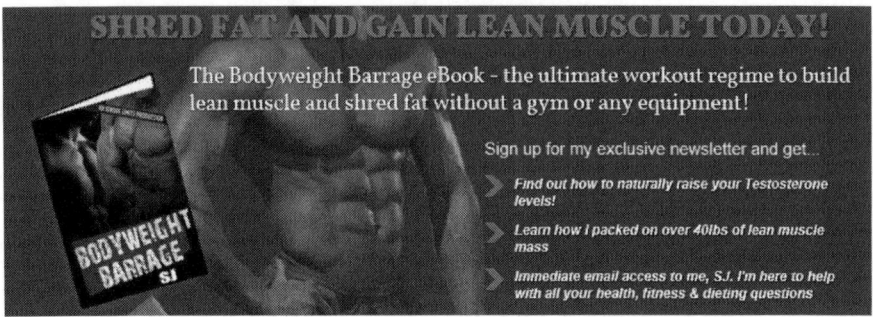

- **The Bodyweight Barrage eBook - the ultimate guide to building muscle and shredding fat without a gym, including exercise descriptions, photos and more!**
- *Immediate email access to me, SJ. Ask me anything, and I'll give you an answer*
- **My honest product reviews and recommendations**

In order to claim your bonus content, simply navigate to:

www.ignorelimits.com/

Enter your email in the box so you can receive this exclusive content instantly!

Chapter 1 - What is Intermittent Fasting?

The simplest and the most accurate definition of Intermittent Fasting (IF) is the alteration of intervals of not eating during the time where you are allowed to eat. IF is a weight loss method that follows the eat-stop-eat pattern that was introduced in 1940. Basically, the process includes a period of fasting, a stage of non-fasting and then you need to fast again. It is an intermittent plan that you need to follow until you have learned how to control your cravings for food and lose your extra weight.

This ebook wants to specify that Intermittent Fasting or IF is not just a diet program. Its primary goal is to promote a better way of life. The idea is on the rise, and lots of health experts have designed their own approach or technique in IF.

From the evolutionary viewpoint, our ancestors fasted during the time when the food was limited or when they were not successful on their hunting trips. So, it is very possible that our bodies are designed to fast occasionally.

Intermittent fasting to lose weight and to improve your health is not a new idea. There are lots of studies on intermittent fasting for the last 18 years. The studies carried out on animals started as early as 1943.

The basic idea of IF is to have a better health through repeated fasting for extended periods as compared to the typical everyday breakfast-lunch-dinner timetable. Disparities are limitless. Some skip breakfast, some prefer to skip dinner. Some people fast all day, every other day, once per week, every third day or once per week.

The different methods of IF will be discussed in the later part of this book, but it is best to mention that the variations in the methods come from extending the fasting window. Normally, the fasting period may vary from sixteen hours up to thirty six hours, and each of those plans has benefits.

You might not know it, but all of us are actually doing some form of fasting. The least technical definition of fasting is simply not eating, so each time you are not eating, you are actually fasting. Most people do not have a structured timetable of meals where there is a continuous fasting, so instead of fasting intermittently, people are doing it haphazardly and there is no better benefit from it.

When you are sleeping, you are fasting. Therefore, you are having fairly rigid fasting for six to eight hours every night until you eat breakfast. This is the reason why the morning meal is called breakfast as you are actually breaking your overnight fast, thus making breakfast as the most essential meal of the day.

The Argument About Breakfast in Intermittent Fasting

Breakfast has an essential role in the intermittent fasting. Actually, it is the main point of argument for individuals looking at IF from the outside. The big question now is, do we really need to eat breakfast?

Supporters of intermittent fasting would probably say no. This contradicts what most dietician and MDs recommend. For many years, people have been made to believe that breakfast is the most vital meal of the day. Actually, there are lots of people who are cautioned by their doctors for not eating their breakfast, especially those who want to lose weight.

There is some truth about it, though. A study done in 2008 indicated that those who ate a heavy breakfast rich in calories, shed more weight as compared to those who didn't. The theory for the outcome was that the higher caloric intake in the morning led people to snack less and decreased overall caloric intake.

The importance of that study was contested for many reasons, one is that in spite the fact that around 90% of Americans eat breakfast, there are still lots of Americans who are overweight. If the first step to weight loss is eating breakfast, then there is something wrong with the process.

There are lots of evidences that support the idea about breakfast. Some epidemiological studies show a connection between a higher body weight and skipping breakfast.

Supporters of the breakfast theory believe that most people are eating the wrong breakfast. This explains why 50% of Americans are overweight. Quick and easy meals such as doughnuts and danishes can result in weight gain.

However, the bottom line of the breakfast study is that a heavy breakfast leads to a minimal overall caloric intake. That is the argument for a heavy breakfast; it boils down to energy balance. The composition of the food shouldn't matter if the weight loss comes down to calories in versus calories out.

The real reason why you need to eat breakfast is insulin sensitivity. In simple terms, the more sensitive your body is to insulin, the more likely you will gain muscle and lose fat. Increasing insulin sensitivity will result in more effective dieting.

The proponents of eating breakfast contend that since insulin sensitivity is elevated in the morning, taking breakfast rich in carbohydrates will ensure the balance of having a huge amount of energy without the risk of weight gain.

This leads to intermittent fasting. Actually, insulin sensitivity is not higher in the morning. It is higher after the eight to ten hour fasting period that you experience when you sleep. Insulin sensitivity is higher when glycogen levels are at a low level, and liver glycogen is at its lowest level when you're sleeping fast.

IF takes it even further. It looks like that lengthening the fasting time beyond that eight to ten hours by not eating breakfast will further increase insulin.

A person can also increase insulin sensitivity in post exercise, thus, in many instances intermittent fasting supporters recommend compounding benefits through training in a fasted state and then taking a carbohydrate rich meal right after your workout.

Basically, this only means that there is nothing special about breakfast, and this explains that if you are fasting intermittently there is no need for you to eat first thing in the morning. You will know when is the best time to eat to break your fast in Chapter 4- Meal Timing.

Before we discuss the Meal timing or frequency, it is important that you know first the benefits of intermittent fasting. This will serve as your driving force to follow the plan and focus your mind on achieving the weight that you want and create a healthy lifestyle.

How to Start with IF

The idea of IF is not what most individuals are willing to do. Depriving oneself of food is not a good idea, particularly if you are hungry. A person feels hungry regularly because the body expects food and the choices available for eating are numerous. Understanding this will enable you to start with IF easily and overcome the few weeks of uncomfortable feeling. Here are some steps that you can use to start intermittent fasting and overcome the first few weeks of unpleasantness.

1. Try it out for one day

IF is no different from other fasting methods. If you consider doing it for the rest of your life, you need to make things easier. On the first day discuss the important things that you need to know and you will discover that it is not that bad to eat only four to eight hours a day. If you try it out for one day, it will be easier for you to move to day two, three and before you know it you are actually fasting normally.

2. Know your goals

Before you start an intermittent fasting protocol, you should know your goals. If your purpose of using it is to lose fat and increase your muscle, then you can carry out a Leangains style (see Chapter 3) 16 hour fast with eight hours feeding window daily. If you choose to do intermittent fasting for disease prevention and anti-aging, you can even get away with 36 hours of fasting. It all depends on your goals, but the remaining under 72 hours is suggested.

3. Time your intermittent fasting for social purposes

Basically, you can do an IF from 9:30 am to 5:30 pm. With this schedule, you will not just eat more meals and calories, but you might cheat more often. Think of social events and the craving to eat dinner later than 5:30pm. It is easier to let yourself to have an 8 hour feeding window from 12pm – 8pm.

4. Drink water when you wake up

The first thing that you need to do when you wake up is to drink water. You might not notice it, but your body is dehydrated while you sleep. Make sure that you replenish the water once you wake up and the feeling of hunger will be dissipated slightly.

5. Fasting is better with coffee/tea

Drinking small amounts of tea will not break the fast, just make sure that there is no extra cream or sugar added. Drink it while it's warm and straight and it will help to focus and eliminate any hunger pangs.

6. You won't crave for food forever

You get hungry every morning when you wake up because you are used to eating every day. After several weeks, you will not get hungry at all while fasting. Within the first week, the hunger should be reduced. Knowing that you will not have to deal with hunger forever is the best way to start from a psychological perspective.

7. Choose a Cheat Day

Some individuals consider it is best to have a cheat day, this means that you can eat whatever foods that you would like. You can choose a day with higher calorie or carbohydrate intake, as well as more sweet potatoes, which are all safer sources to indulge upon.

8. Keep busy while fasting

One of the primary reasons why fasting overnight is easy is because you are asleep. If you are fasting while awake, keep yourself busy as best as you can. If you focus too much on fasting it will not help.

9. Choose the right food

You may discover that the best way to improve your health is through the intermittent fasting, but it will not work if you do not eat the right food during your feeding window.

10.   It is not intended for all

Intermittent fasting is not for everyone. Assess yourself for a few weeks and check if the practice is right for you. Definitely, there are lots of proof that it is a healthy and good practice, but for some individuals, it might not work.

Pregnant or breastfeeding mothers should not fast, as well as those with serious medical conditions. Talk to a doctor if you want to make sure that the process is safe for you.

Intermittent Fasting – A Healthy Option

Eating extra meals can keep your metabolism revved up, making weight loss much simpler. There are, however, some proofs that support this idea, and a good amount of proof that disputes it. For instance, a study published in the British Journal of Nutrition stated that any outcomes of meal pattern in controlling the body weight seem to be negligible, and what is important is the overall food intake.

In practice, those additional meals are not vegetable intensive, home cooked foods. At present, they are known as energy bars, snacks, and others. In short, they are high-glycemic processed snacks.

If people are advised to "eat several small meals," some may interpret this as "eat all the time," which may result in compulsive overeating. There are some Americans who think that if they are eating three meals with no snacks, it is a form of intermittent fasting.

The basic idea of intermittent fasting is to enjoy a healthy lifestyle by fasting repeatedly for longer periods as compared to the typical daily breakfast-lunch-dinner pattern.

Chapter 2 - Benefits of Intermittent Fasting

There are several benefits that you can enjoy with intermittent fasting that make it so popular. Those who practice IF eat less frequently. Aside from feeling hungry less often and getting easily full when they eat, these individuals benefit in terms of logistics and practicality.

Since you will eat less, you will prepare or buy fewer meals. As a result, you can save your money and time. This also means that you will be exposed to flavors less often and thus you are less likely to get bored and eat food that you shouldn't.

Also, by eating less frequently, you will eat less calories.

Included in the IF plan is a full-day fasting that reduces the calorie intake drastically. If you are applying the 24 hours twice per week (See Chapter 4 for details.), you are actually reducing your food intake by about 30%. It is not difficult to see how that would result in weight loss.

Here are some essential benefits of intermittent fasting:

Longevity

You want to get healthy so you can live longer. Longevity will open you up to the opportunity to experience more in life. You will have more time for your family, learning more, and enjoying life. But people are familiar with the idea that to live longer, you should eat less. You probably grew up with the idea that each time you take something unhealthy, you are actually causing harm to your own body. This is not the case with intermittent fasting. Eating the food you want from time to time is not prohibited.

One of the studies done in IF way back in 1940 made use of rats as their test subjects. The group who conducted the study were able to prove that IF will not affect the natural growth of the rats. Also, it lengthened their lifespan.

Another part of this research shows that by limiting calorie intake, there is a reduction in insulin in the brain that will lead to longer life.

Detoxification

We are exposed to many toxins and we will be exposed to even more toxins in the future. Of the 30,000 toxins that are being used by many individuals on a daily basis, only 3,500 of these are safe. It is impossible to avoid these toxins. Anywhere we go, we are exposed to toxins. We get it from the air, via our skin and from the food we eat. This is one of the reasons why there are lots of modern illnesses like nervous system disorders, cancer, birth defects, and diabetes.

Detoxification is the process of controlling the body's ability to excrete toxins. In fact, your body detoxifies 24/7. It is a continuous task. However, if you have a poor diet, the process is delayed. If you practice IF, you give your body enough time to replenish as it focuses on its cellular custodial tasks. It centers on cleansing. A study about the relation of intermittent fasting to Huntington's and Alzheimer's diseases showed that when detoxification is at its optimum during a fast, it lowers a person's risk of having the said degenerative diseases. The limitation in your food intake that IF provides promotes neurogenesis. As you fast, your brain is going through maintenance, making your brain become stronger.

Weight Loss

There are lots of people who are struggling with their weight despite the many helpful dietary solutions out there. Each time you eat, the sugars you consume are stored in the liver as glycogen. Once your glycogen storage is full, the excess sugar will be stored as fat. Glycogen is the first source of energy when it comes to your everyday activities. Your body is like a car, and glycogen will serve as the fuel for your body. After taking a meal, your body won't require new glycogen until seven to eight hours afterward. It only means that your body will be able to function properly, even if you fast. Once you used up all your stored glycogen, your body will depend on your stored fat as a source of energy. This is where weight loss will take place.

Intermittent fasting will force your body to use your stored fats. If you fast longer, the more weight you will lose.

Hormone Regulation

HGH or Human Growth Hormone is one of the essential hormones that keep you looking young. This is the reason why lots of pharmaceutical companies produce products that will boost the HGH production within the pituitary glands. Most of these supplements are being abused by many and there are many harmful side effects when you overuse the product. If you practice intermittent fasting, you will be able to boost the production of this hormone. A study has shown that IF, when combined with exercise, increased the production of HGH in women by 1300% and 2000% in men.

Leptin

Leptin is the hormone responsible in turning off the hunger switch of your body when you achieved the amount of fat that is enough for reproduction and survival. This is also one of the primary reasons why low fat diets are not effective. If you don't eat fat or if you consume only a small amount of fat, you will still feel hungry and you will end up gaining weight rather than losing it.

Overweight individuals have high levels of Leptin. Ironically, their brain sends a message to stop eating, but the body is deaf to these signals, causing them to gain weight. This will lead to overproduction of Leptin, which takes place when there is lots of fat in the body. IF will let the body regulate Leptin back to normal levels, which makes it more effective as a hunger regulating hormone.

Diabetes

For illnesses like diabetes, one of the most essential factors is insulin resistance. Because of the abundance of modern food, it is easy to increase blood sugar levels. In doing so, our hormones will be completely out of balance. Problems with insulin are definitely the cause of most diabetes associated problems. In a study carried out in Berkeley, CA, calorie restriction and a form of IF was tested on animals and came up with startling conclusions.

During the analysis, fasting glucose levels decreased. Several studies showed a decrease in glucose concentrations after twenty to twenty four weeks. In simple terms, the test animals were able to control the sugar level to avoid diabetes.

Cardiovascular Disorder

Poor cardiovascular performance is the outcome of poor lifestyle factors, like inadequte exercise and dieting. Two of the leading factors in cardiovascular disease are clogged arteries and elevated cholesterol levels, most of the time directed towards a brewing storm. A study conducted at the University of Utah asked 500 individuals who had fasted one day per month and discovered that they were 40% less likely to have clogged arteries. Also, after 3 weeks of IF protocols, patients were able to enjoy increased HDL levels and reduced triglyceride levels. The effect on blood pressure in humans has not been seen, but is apparent in animals. For people with the proper dietary regimen, clogging of arteries seems to be less of a problem.

Anti-Aging

The study done concerning aging and caloric restriction is clear, but who wants to eat less? With IF you can enjoy the many benefits that you can also get from caloric restriction, but you can still eat more of what you want.

One of the primary factors in aging is oxidative stress, and IF can reduce the damage to your cells. The evidence shows that IF decreases the markers of oxidative stress while increasing the levels of the anti-oxidants in the body.

Hormones play an essential role in aging. Insulin-like growth factor promotes reproduction and growth, but this quickens aging. With decreased IGF-1 from IF, your body starts to repair cells.

Through intermittent fasting, oxidative stress is reduced without the need to lower calorie intake.

Lifestyle Change

One of the important benefits people can get from intermittent fasting is the freedom from eating all day long. Many people are trapped from eating at specific times, constantly worrying about food and eating all day long. It will make your life much easier since you don't have to worry a lot about the food you need to eat. This is the outcome if you accept that something so simple can actually work for you.

Chapter 3 - Styles of Intermittent Fasting

It looks like that over the past 15 to 20 years, thousands of diet books have been printed and they are all different. Actually, lots of them have been in direct opposition to each other.

In spite of the different nature of these diets, the one thing that has been consistently suggested in most diet books published is the frequency of meals. If you have read a diet book, hired a personal trainer or seen a nutritionist you have probably been told that to lose weight, you need to eat 5 to 6 small meals per day.

The style of eating also known as the frequent feeding model, is popular with everyone from dietitians to bodybuilders and has been practiced most of the time for so long that it is usually taken as fact.

There are several styles of intermittent fasting, some of the popular styles are as follows:

24 Hour Fast

This style entails going 24 hours without food. This implies that if your last food intake was at 6pm today, then you should not eat until 6pm the next day. However, you are allowed to drink lots of calorie-free beverages.

Very simple to use, and easy to follow compared to other Intermittent fasting methods – you don't eat for 24 hours once or twice a week. You can drink water freely and other non-caloric beverages while fasting. After the 24 hours fast, you will eat a regular meal. The best way to eat after fasting is to pretend as if you didn't fast. Make sure that you don't overeat, just eat a regular meal.

This style of intermittent fasting is very effective and can be proven by several individuals who have used this style.

It is flexible. For individuals who prefer this method of IF, it is highly recommended that they fast during their busiest days. By doing this, you don't focus on not eating and potential hunger, but rather you can be very productive. Also, in case you will be having a family event or other social gathering coming, you can change the dates of your fasting days.

Lots of health benefits. Aside from fat loss there are lots of health benefits as mentioned in Chapter 2. This method is very easy to follow. There is no need for you to count calories, limit your favorite foods or weigh food. It only means that you can eat any food that you want to eat.

For some people, this process could be too difficult – there are some who are having a hard time going to extended period of time without eating. There are some who experience headache, get cranky, too anxious or get fatigued. For those who are having some difficulties, breaking in to fasting, and go as long as you can in the early part and slowly increase the fasting phase over time.

For some individuals using the 24hour method leads to binge eating – even if you need to eat a normal meal after the fast, some individuals think they are allowed to eat anything and they consider it as a reward for fasting for 24 hours.

The Leangains Method – 14-16 Hours Daily Fast

This type of intermittent fasting is promoted by famous IF guru Martin Berkhan. He has carried out a lot of research on this method, and there are lots of people who are getting the result that they want.

Women fast for 14 hours and men fast for 16 hours. For instance, if your last meal is at 8pm tonight, you should not eat again until 10am if you are a woman and 12pm if you are a man.

As with 24 hours fast method of intermittent fasting, you don't eat any food or caloric beverages while fasting. Sugar free gum, water and other non-caloric beverages are allowed. As compared to 14-16 hours daily fast, you need to skip breakfast. For some individuals this could be quite hard at first, particularly if they believed that breakfast is the most important meal of the day. Some individuals may feel sick, light headed or sluggish if they don't eat breakfast.

It is best to eat three meals a day without taking any snacks in between, but consuming two large meals is also fine. Since you will only be eating 3 or 2 times a day, you will be eating larger meals and it only means that you will feel full.

If you have a social life this method is much easier to follow, because you can eat larger meals, it is easier to go to social gatherings and restaurants without the need to stress yourself about what you are going to eat.

This type of IF can be used to build muscle, fat loss and even maintenance, so it is adaptable for any goal.

The Warrior Diet – The Daily 20-ish Hour Partial Fast

This type of IF is created by Ori Hofmekler. With this method you need to perform a 20-ish hour partial fast daily, and then have one huge meal at night.

During the fasting part of the day, you can eat some few servings of raw vegetables and fruits, fresh veggie/fruit juices, and some servings of protein if desired. These are limited. You take your main meal at night. This style includes lists of food to eat and when to eat certain foods.

Some of the Ori's recommendations are quite strict and can be hard to follow long term, but some people were able to follow it.

Consuming such a large meal at night may not work for everyone. There are some people who are comfortable feeling full after eating such a large meal. But, some people love it.

It can be hard to get in all of your veggies, protein, and fruits with just one large meal.

You might bring on the wrong foods. Some individuals will inevitably think that they have eaten hardly anything the entire day, so they can eat anything that they want at night. Then they will end up eating only wings, pizza and cookies every night.

There is no need for you to worry about food all day. For many, this is the best benefit of the Warrior Diet. Since you eat a large meal at night, there is no need to worry about preparing food during the day.

It saves a lot of money and time. Since you won't be eating that much, so most likely, you will save some money on your food bill. Also, you don't have to spend some time preparing your food.

Boost energy levels – there are lots of people who tend to experience greater energy levels when fasting.

This method is best suited if you want to lose fat and not to build muscle mass. Others may have a different result.

If you work around social gatherings that take place during daytime, you might have a hard time.

Fat Loss Forever IF Method

This method is the combination of the most well known methods of intermittent fasting – Eat Stop Eat, Leangins and The Warrior Diet. Dan Go and John Romaniello have created a hybrid fasting method that combined all the popular methods in the most sophisticated and intelligent way, all for one purpose – to utilize the strengths of every method to cancel out the weaknesses of others and created their own method known as Fat Loss Forever.

Aside from the combination of the 3 intermittent fasting methods discussed above, they likewise include a Roman method termed Feast/Fast. In a nutshell, this type of IF includes an entire cheat day followed by a thirty six hour fast.

Here are some important facts about Fat Loss Forever. This method is intended to do 2 things:

1. Offer a twelve week program that will aid in burning fat quicker.

2. Aid in maintaining the outcome for your entire lifetime – via the great benefits of IF – by giving you the simplest nutrition lifestyle ever made.

What are the possible drawbacks of FLF? First, if you don't do well with IF, then you won't like this. Likewise, you have a particular intermittent fasting method to follow on specific days, and that, for some people, could be confusing or very challenging. Others may eat too much during the cheat days and eat lots of processed and trans-fat laden junk. If you do not handle cheat days properly, then this could not be the method for you.

5:2 Diet Plan

This type of intermittent fasting is very simple. All you need to do is to limit yourself to 500 calories a day if you are a woman and 600 calories if you are a man for two non-consecutive days a week. This idea of the 5:2 diet works by putting your body into repair mode instead of starvation mode or storing fat, which can take place when you simply cut down all together. This repair mode will help the body restore damaged cells, which utilizes more energy.

The structure of this diet is very simple – for any two days of the week, you should eat fewer calories. The fasting days can be any day from Monday to Friday to fit a busy lifestyle. Because the duration of each fasting day is quickly over and it is best to enjoy food with friends and family during non-fast days, this method to weight management is said to be sustained by the majority of people who tested it.

The short fasting would put the body into a metabolic state that will trigger recovery and repair at the cellular level. This affects several hormones and gives the digestive system, and other organs, some time to rest, particularly the pancreas, the gland which generates insulin in response to sugar and carbohydrates. This helps the body to be more sensitive to insulin, which is one of the most essential aspects of not just weight loss but also lowering the risk of diabetes.

Secondly, by having short term fasts, they have a better sense of control over what they eat during the non-fast days, rarely eat out of boredom and have a tendency to select foods which are healthier.

The first fasting days can be difficult, but upon getting used to how it feels to have a sense of hunger, there are some people that think that their fasts days are enjoyable. There are some that feel lighter, more energetic, more alert and awake. It is important that the 5:2 diet is dealt sensibly. Because of the fasting days, it is not a diet that is recommended for anyone who has an eating disorder. The fasts days should include the recommended amount of the calories and the non-fast days should not be calorie restricted to make sure that over the week you will still consume sufficient amount of calories.

Chapter 4 - Meal Timing

If you search online, you will get confused with the advice that you will find about optimal meal frequency. As mentioned in Chapter 1, breakfast jump-starts fat burning and eating five to six small meals a day can boost metabolism.

Modern wisdom dictates that breakfast is important, it boosts your metabolism for the day and aids in losing weight.

Observational studies show that skipping breakfast are more likely to make people obese as compared to those who eat breakfast. But it is not a proven fact that breakfast can help you lose weight, its eating breakfast that reduces the risk of being obese. Experts suggest that if you are hungry when you wake up, you can eat breakfast. If not, don't... ensure that you will eat healthy foods for the rest of the day.

Eating More Frequent Meals Boost Metabolism

The concept of eating smaller meals more frequently to boost metabolism is a continuing myth. It is a fact that consuming a meal slightly boosts metabolism and this phenomenon is known as the TEF or the thermic effect of food.

However, it is the total food intake that determines the amount of energy used during digestion. Eating three meals of 800 calories will result to the same thermic effect as eating six meals of 400 calories. Actually, there is no difference. Several studies have compared fewer, larger meals vs many smaller meals and concluded that there is no greater impact on either total amount of fat loss or metabolic rate.

Eating More Frequently to Balance Blood Sugar Levels and Reduce Cravings

To balance the blood sugar levels, people should eat more often. Some people do not agree on this, but scientifically it is true. Taking big meals may lead to faster rise and fall in blood sugar, while consuming smaller, more frequent meals can help normalize blood sugar levels throughout the day. However, this fast is not supported by science.

Several studies prove that those who eat less larger meals have lower blood glucose levels on average. They may have bigger spikes in blood sugar, but all in all their levels are much lower. This is very important for individuals with blood sugar issues, because high blood sugars will result in different types of issues.

Eating less frequent will also result to improve satiety and reduce hunger than eating more frequent meals.

Eating Frequent Meals May Cause Colon Cancer

Some observational studies show that more frequent eating is associated with increased risk of colon cancer, which is known as the fourth most common cause of cancer death. The risk is higher for four meals a day, around 90% as compared to two meals.

Correlation does not equal causation. Therefore, these studies are not enough to prove that eating frequent meals increases the risk of having colon cancer.

The Health Benefits of Skipping Meals From Time to Time

A very hot topic in nutrition these days is intermittent fasting – which is defined in Chapter 1 as not eating at certain times like skipping breakfast and lunch and then taking a full meal after several hours of fasting.

Based on the modern wisdom, this method would put you in starvation mode and you will lose some muscle mass. But, this is not the case.

Studies show that on short-term fasting metabolism is increased at the start. The metabolic rate goes down, only after two to three days.

Also, studies in both animals and humans show that IF has several health benefits as discussed in Chapter 2. IF also induces a cellular cleanup process known as autophagy, where the body eliminates that buildup in the cells and contributes to disease and aging.

Chapter 5 - Supplementation when Fasting

Here is a list of supplements that you may find helpful depending on your goals. The first four supplements on the list provide more benefits to the users. Adding these supplements to the healthy food that you eat is the best way to safeguard against any possible shortcomings of a repetitive diet. Other supplements will help with fat loss, performance or can make life easier. They are not essential by any means.

Multivitamins

Taking multivitamins together with your first meal is a cheap and simple way to safeguard yourself against any possible mineral and vitamin deficiencies in your diet. This is not necessary, but it is better to be safe than sorry.

Omega-3 Fatty Acids or Fish Oil

Having a good omega 3-to-omega 6 ratio is vital. Taking 2g EPA and 1.5g DHA every day is enough to get those muscles grow.

Calcium

Calcium boosts testosterone levels and increases fat excretion. Taking a 500-750 mg tablet of calcium with your everyday diet will help you with your goals. However, if you get enough calcium from your diet, there is no need to add more.

Vitamin D

Some scientific evidence suggests that there are lots of people who do not get the right amount of Vitamin D to perform well. Some medical breakthroughs get interested for this vitamin and some of its benefits. Vitamin D can actually boost strength and athletic performance. A daily intake of Vitamin D at 2000

IU/day is a safe and conservative dosage, but some individuals use higher doses without any negative effects.

Amino Acids

The amino acids aid with intra-set recovery and muscle endurance in the higher rep ranges. Take 10g pre-workout, during fasting.

Creatine

This is the only legal supplement with several scientific studies that support its effectiveness. The creatine elevates the muscle for a direct performance boost. It boosts muscle growth through effects on satellite cell proliferation, insulin-like growth factor-1 signaling and myogenic transcription factors.

Beta-Alanine

Beta-Alanine is an amino acid that can stand alone and can boost exercise performance. It improves performance during single bouts of exercise that last more than 60 seconds and multiple bouts of high-intensity exercise. Thus, it won't improve your optimum strength, but anaerobic threshold and time to exhaustion will be improved.

Whey Protein

This is perfect during post and pre workout. It is best to use 100% Whey. It has the ability to increase HGH. One of the benefits of intermittent fasting is that it increases the hormone known HGH, adding whey protein in your diet will definitely boost the production of this hormone.

Casein Protein

You can use this supplement any time of the day, but the ideal time of taking this is during pre-bedtime. This is slow releasing and provides more satiety as compared to whey protein.

Glucosamine

Glucosamine is safe and is an effective supplement for relieving pain and stiffness in joints.

For fat loss, keep in mind that IF boosts the effect of stimulants. Any stimulant that you take during the fasted period will have a greater effect as compared to its ingestion during the feeding stage. Caution should be exercised for those who are not familiar with the utilization of stimulants.

Caffeine

If you are not a coffee drinker, you are missing out by not including caffeine in your diet. It is cheap, suppress appetite and has thermogenic properties.

Chapter 6 - Popularity of Intermittent Fasting

Intermittent fasting is one of the powerful interventions that shed excess weight and lower your risk of chronic diseases such as heart disease and diabetes. These health benefits are more or less beneficial side effects of altering your body from burning sugar to eliminating fat as its fuel. Because it is very effective and it provides lots of benefits, intermittent fasting now gets more mainstream media attention.

Recently, The Wall Street Journal posted an article about intermittent calorie restriction, particularly the 5:2 diet, endorsed by Dr. Michael Mosley in his book The Fast Diet.

The 5:2 method involves eating 5 days a week regularly, and fasting for 2 days. During the fasting days, Dr. Mosley suggests reducing your food intake to ¼ of your regular daily calories, or around 500 calories for women and 600 calories for men, together with lots of tea and water.

The article from The Wall Street Journal mentioned that some research shows that this radical approach may be difficult to implement at first, but as you go along, it becomes easier compared to the usual route of lowering calories each day. Some studies done in animals suggest it also offers other health benefits which include cognitive improvements.

Another popular news portal New York Daily News posted an article about intermittent fasting, states that it is the biggest diet craze. Also in this news the writer describes intermittent fasting as a trend that shows no sign of going away. It is rapidly becoming the hottest diet trends.

CBS News posted an article (April 4, 2014) about the study conducted by Dr. Krista Varandy, an assistant professor of kinesiology and nutrition at the University of Illinois, who developed the intermittent fasting diet that's working for people like Green. She noticed that intermittent fasters eat only 10% more than they actually need in a standard diet during the non-fasting days, which is less than what a lot of people eat. At present, Varandy is carrying out a year long study, funded by the National Institutes of Health, in which participants follow an intermittent fasting plan for 6 months and then a higher calorie diet for the next six months. The primary purpose of the study is to check whether or not intermittent fasting is an effective tool for weight maintenance.

Reasons Why Intermittent Fasting is Very Effective

One of the main mechanisms that makes IF so beneficial for health is associated with its effect on your insulin sensitivity. Sugar is the primary source of energy for your body. It also promotes insulin resistance when taken in the quantity found in the modern processed food diets. The primary driver of chronic disease from heart disease to cancer is insulin resistance. The risk of chronic disease is reduced when the body becomes accustomed to burning fat instead of sugar as its primary fuel. Becoming fat adapted could be the key strategy for both cancer prevention and treatment, as cancer cells cannot use fat for fuel – they need sugar to succeed.

Fasting increases insulin sensitivity together with mitochondrial energy efficiency, thus delaying aging and disease, which are usually related to loss of insulin sensitivity and reduced mitochondrial energy. The two additional mechanisms in which fasting benefits your body is:

Reducing Oxidative Stress

Intermittent fasting reduces the buildup of oxidative radicals in the cells, and thus preventing oxidative damage to lipids, cellular proteins, and nucleic acids—the same damage that is a factor in aging and in susceptibility to diseases.

Increasing capacity to resist disease, aging and stress – fasting stimulates a cellular stress response in which cells up-regulate the gene expressions that increase the capacity to deal with stress and resist aging and disease.

Cravings Vanish Instantly as Excess Weight Falls Off

IF has been proven to be as the most effective way to eliminate excess weight. This could be challenging in the beginning, but as soon as you have adapted to eliminating fat, you will notice that sugar cravings vanish without a trace.

Studies Conducted to Prove the Effectiveness of Intermittent Fasting

The popularity of intermittent fasting is increasing. Because of this, studies are carried out both in humans and in animals to test the effectiveness of the said approach.

The First Fasts

Religions believed that fasting is good for the soul, but its benefits on the body were not widely recognized until the 1900s, when the doctors started to recommend it to help cure several disorders – like obesity, epilepsy and diabetes.

A study on calorie limitation performed in the 1930s, after nutritionist Clive McCay of Cornell University discovered that rats that had undergone daily fasting from an early stage of their lives live longer, and were less likely to have cancer as well as other diseases as they aged, than rats that ate at will. A study on calorie restriction and intermittent fasting intersected in 1945, when University of Chicago scientists reported an alternate-day feeding lengthens the life span of rats as much as daily dieting in McCay's previous experiments.

Also, IF seems to delay the development of the disease that lead to death, this is based on the research done by University of Chicago.

In the next years research into anti aging diets took a back seat to more powerful medical advances, like the continued development of antibiotics and coronary artery bypass surgery. Mattson along with other researchers have supported the idea that intermittent fasting reduces the risks of degenerative brain diseases in later life. Mattson and his group have shown that episodic fasting keeps neurons protected against several types of damaging stress, at least in rats.

One of the earliest studies showed that alternate-day feeding made the rats' brains resistant to toxins that promote cellular damage to the type of cells last as they age. In a follow up study, Mattson and his group discovered that IF protects rats against stroke damage, controls motor deficits in a rat model of Parkinson's disease and slows cognitive decline in mice genetically engineered to copy the symptoms of Alzheimer's.

Mattson tested IF and skipped breakfast and lunch except on weekends. According to him it makes him more productive. Mattson, a 55 year old Ph.D holder in biology, thinks that IF acts in part as a form of mild stress that revs up cellular protections against molecular damage.

Research done by Valter Longo at the University of Southern California Longevity Institute conclude that IF has a beneficial effect on IGF-1, an insulin like growth factor that plays an essential role in aging. If you eat, this hormone helps your cells to reproduce, and while this is ideal for growth, it is also a factor that boosts the aging process. IF decreases the IGF-1 expression, and changes in other DNA repair genes. In this process, intermittent fasting controls your body from growth mode to repair mode.

Research by Mark Hartman and his group indicates short-term fasting can activate the production of HGH or Human Growth Hormone in men, and reduce oxidative stress that contributes to aging and disease. Benefits brain health, clarity of thought and mental well-being.

Chapter 7 - Cons of Intermittent Fasting

Periodic fasting is very popular these days. Just like other diet regimen, it is not surprising that there are downsides to the regimen that will make it a passing fancy in both the general and fitness population. The use of intermittent eating patterns to get rid of fat can be effective, but that does not mean it is healthy, can be sustained for a long time, or will benefit athletes.

Non-experts and experts in the field of fitness and nutrition recommend a variety of fasting methods or meal frequency – fasting every 16 hours, all day, every 20 hours, twice a week, every third day, every other day, once a week, or just when you are not hungry. The definition of fasting differs – In some instances, it means eating berries and green vegetables when fasting. Some take oatmeal and protein-carb drinks are recommended.

At present, many religions / cultures use fasting as a spiritual practice, but, in the animal world, no animal is known to voluntarily fast unless it is not feeling well. In most instances, the same animal will eat plants to promote vomiting.

The study done on animal on intermittent fasting is in no way conclusive, but trends on showing that it is very beneficial for the men's health- reproduction is enhanced – but is not safe for women – they become infertile. For instance, stop menstruating, female rats masculinize, they become hyperactive, and sleep less. The researchers discovered that when the rats bodies sense a starvation state, rats generate traits that will aid them to find food.

The same trends are reported by humans who have tested intermittent fasting. Researches and personal reports of women and men suggest the following cons to the practice:

- Craving for food during the fast period (monitoring the time in anticipation of the next meal, which lead to anxiety).

- An over dependence on coffee that lead to severe adrenal fatigue, circadian dysregulation and hormonal.

- Insomnia, specifically among women, due to the hypocretin neurons activation that incite wakefulness.

- Over time, the ovaries shut down and women stay awake at night, probably an adaptive response so they can look for food to keep them alive. In short, why become pregnant if you are going to starve the baby?

- Hormonal havoc for women takes several forms, which includes adult acne, obsession over body image, menstrual irregularities and metabolic disturbance.

For athletes, and those who are interested in building muscle mass or are engaged in living energetic lifestyles, fasting is not recommended due to following reasons:

1. **Optimum Physical and Cognitive Performance Needs Regular Nourishings**

   The apparent and biggest issue of infrequent nourishing is twofold:

   a) Acute hormonal deregulation that will result to poor energy, focus and altered homeostasis,

   b) If you lack amino acids in the blood, it will cause a catabolic effect on muscle.

Initially, reports suggest that intermittent fasting improves brain function, insulin health, and enhances alertness, especially in men. The effects seem to be negative for women, and the long term impact for men, particularly lean men who are into athletic performance, are suboptimal.

Simply, eating irregularly results in erratic blood sugar and spikes in insulin. Basically, neurotransmitters, circadian rhythms and hormones get out of whack. By following the Paleo diet of high-protein, low-carb, healthy fat, you can activate the energetic brain transmitters and the hypocretin neurons by nourishing the body rather than starving it. This provides a continuous source of amino acids for building muscle and boosts metabolism and cognition.

By consuming a high-protein, healthy fat meal, low-carb every few hours, you can boost the energizing pathways in the body for optimum brain function and energy levels. This provides a balanced blood sugar, a strong but flexible homeostasis for longevity and better insulin signalling.

2. Protein Synthesis for Muscle Building Needs Protein Nourishing

There is a great variation between adding muscle and not losing muscle. If you don't provide the body with the right amount of protein every few hours, muscle deterioration will take place. Surely, there are some that will argue that you can maintain muscle by applying an intermittent eating pattern, but there are some that is more interested in boosting optimal muscle mass for performance and health. The good thing is that there are lots of studies done about this issue. Here are some of the studies done:

Positive muscle protein synthesis to increase muscle tissue needs some stimuli, including anabolic hormones, amino acids and a high degree of tension from weight training. For instance, a 2010 study on active, but underweight men on a calorie restricted diet that provided strong dose 1.5g/kg/bw of protein a day resulted in a 20% reduction of protein synthesis after ten days. The outcome was a one kilogram loss of muscle.

An example of the advantages of eating frequent meals is a study in which trained young men carried out a lower body workout and then consume 80gms of protein in one of three protein dosing patterns – eight ten gram doses every one hour and thirty minutes, four twenty gram doses every three hours, or two forty gram doses every six hours. Those who take thirty grams of protein every three hours had greater protein synthesis and an increased protein balance as compared to other feeding plans.

Another study that supports the continuous protein feeding showed how young men who took forty grams of protein before bedtime boost protein synthesis by twenty five percent – an amazing amount. The men carried out his training at night, then took protein at 11:30 pm and protein synthesis was continued all night.

As compared to short-term muscle loss with infrequent feedings is seen in a three day human study in which young men take their meal twice a day with twelve hour intervals. The men experienced much greater use of muscle protein for energy as compared to a group with five meals. The researchers caution against the use of irregular meal frequencies, especially in older people, because it will increase the decline in sarcopenia and muscle mass. The balance between protein loss and protein building, which is over time would result in a loss of muscle mass, is very delicate. If you neglect or forget to feed the body in regular doses during the 24 hour period after weight training, the protein synthesis will be reduced and there is a delay in recovery.

3. Intermittent Fasting Could Lead to Adrenal Stress

The impact of the long-term toll of eating patterns and the short-term dietary change that go against circadian rhythms is very different. IF continued for a few weeks or a month will not lead to adrenal fatigue for extended period, but that doesn't imply that it is the appropriate way to change the body composition.

The short-term effect on performance is small but is important in a study that tested how Ramadan IF affected fatigue and performance in judo athletes. Results show that daytime fasting would lead to intense feelings of fatigue, a decrease in anaerobic performance and power output, and a loss of 1.8% body mass of which 0.65 kg fat lost.

There have been no studies carried out concerning long-term effects of irregular eating in athletes, but the outcome can be predicted based on what you know about overtraining. Fasting for a long period of time will increase the catecholamine hormones. If you are doing this day in and day out, it can lead to adrenal glands fatigue and will cause shutdown. The

41

adrenal hormone receptors will be less responsive that leads to chronic exhaustion, altered metabolism, and reduced central   nervous   drive.

Short term IF will decrease the athletic performance. Long-term will result to adrenal fatigue and lack of homeostasis in the body.

4. Insulin Health Is More Concerned About What You Eat than When to Eat

Erratic eating habits affect blood sugar and insulin health. The study is not conclusive on this issue – men may improve insulin health, for women it is worse. The fat in both genders may improve insulin health, but other factors are influenced such as blood pressure, and fasting, like caloric restriction, is considered by many scientists unsustainable.

However, don't believe that intermittent fasting improves insulin sensitivity. A study in the journal PLOS One compared glucose and insulin over three days in response to an IF model and regular meals five times a day using a diet of 55% carbs, 30% fat and 15% protein. This study showed that IF generate greater spikes and troughs of glucose and insulin, which indicates a biological milieu primed for insulin resistance over time.

Restricting high-glycemic carbs is important to insulin and blood sugar health. A study carried out to compare eating 3 high-carb, 6 high-protein low carb or 6 high-carb meals a day discovered that blood sugar was highest during the 6-carb meals, next is the 3-carb meals, while the insulin was the same in both carb models. The high-protein meals lower glucose and insulin levels dramatically.

For insulin health, give importance to what you eat—particularly good fat, protein, and low-glycemic carbs—instead on when you eat.

5. Intermittent Fasting May Mess Up Circadian Rhythms and Hormones

The impact of IF on circadian rhythm and hormones is devastating. First, the hormonal cascade – anabolic hormones such as growth hormone and testosterone, metabolic hormones like insulin, and energizing hormones of the adrenal glands – is interrelated. If one hormone-producing becomes out of control, you can be sure that others will be affected negatively.

This can result in infertility, poor metabolism and body composition, sleep disorders, increased risk of disease, inability to build muscle, chronic fatigue, and a pro-inflammatory state.

A peek of this with IF comes from an eight-week study in which middle-aged individuals went on a one-meal-a-day diet or a regular three meal a day diet calories were not limited. The results showed that one meal a day group diet have shed off 2 kg of fat as compared to the three meals a day group, but it also resulted to increase in blood pressure. An increase in blood pressure indicates that the circadian rhythms is altered.

Also, cortisol, which was measured in the afternoon before taking the one meal, was 48% lower than at baseline. Diurnal dysregulation is also observed. Definitely, you want to control cortisol for health and body composition, but that does not necessarily mean you want irregular cortisol, which is a sign of adrenal fatigue.

The result is that the reduced meal frequency does not afford significant health benefits for humans.

Intermittent fasting can lead to fat loss, but it is not the best approach. Actually, it might put you at risk of altering circadian rhythms and your hormones. Your body's ability to control itself might be compromised that might lead to disease and exhaustion.

Conclusion

The information provided in this ebook on how to carry out intermittent fasting effectively will help you achieve the results that you want. Because this method works and is supported by science and the personal experiences of those who practice it successfully, expert body builders, health professionals, nutritionist and others recommend this.

Although we are aware that not all calories are created equal, limiting your calorie intake has an essential role in weight loss. If you fast, you are also making it easier to limit your calorie intake over the course of the week. This will give your body the chance to lose weight as you are simply eating less calories than you were consuming in the past.

Intermittent fasting simplifies your day. Instead of having to prepare, eat, pack and time your meals every two to three hours, you can skip a meal or two and just worry about eating food in your eating window.

Intermittent fasting also requires less time. Instead of having to purchase or prepare 3 to 6 meals a day, you only require to prepare two meals. Instead of pausing what you are doing six times a day to eat, you only need to stop to eat twice. Instead of having to do the dishes 6 times, you only have to do them twice. Instead of having to purchase six meals a day, you only need to buy two.

It increases growth hormone secretion, and promotes stronger insulin sensitivity, two important factors for muscle gain and weight loss. This was explained in the chapter 2, but IF helps you create a double whammy for weight loss.

Men and women will have different results, each person will have different results. The best way to find out is to test it on your own.

If this seems that this practice will fit you, then give it a shot. If it sounds crazy to you, find out why you think it sounds crazy, and discover it on your own by experimenting before condemning it.

If you are wondering why others are getting the best results and have changed their lives tremendously through intermittent fasting, maybe it is time for you to apply the approach and find it out on your own.

If you enjoyed this book be sure to check out the tons of great content I post on my blog, it contains everything from fitness and dieting to motivation and brain training. www.ignorelimits.com

Appendix (referenced Studies & Information)

How Intermittent Fasting Might Help You Live a Longer and Healthier Life, Dec 2012

http://www.scientificamerican.com/article/how-intermittent-fasting-might-help-you-live-longer-healthier-life/?page=2

Evidence for Programmed Age, 2009

http://www.programmed-aging.org/theory-3/longo.html

http://mljohnson.pharm.virginia.edu/pdfs/167.pdf

Lean Gains Top Ten Fasting Myths Debunked, Martin Berkhan, Nov 2010
http://www.leangains.com/2010/10/top-ten-fasting-myths-debunked.html

Department of Medicine, University of Rochester School of Medicine and Dentistry, NY, Oct 1987 Leucine, glucose, and energy metabolism after 3 days of fasting in healthy human subjects
http://www.ncbi.nlm.nih.gov/pubmed/3661473

24236303R20032

Made in the USA
San Bernardino, CA
17 September 2015